Otília J. de Carvalho Neta
Kamana B. R. Basílio de Sousa
Fabio C. L. Nepomuceno

Chronic obstructive pulmonary disease

Otília J. de Carvalho Neta
Kamana B. R. Basílio de Sousa
Fabio C. L. Nepomuceno

Chronic obstructive pulmonary disease

Anatomo-clinical approach and its pulmonary involvement

ScienciaScripts

Imprint

Any brand names and product names mentioned in this book are subject to trademark, brand or patent protection and are trademarks or registered trademarks of their respective holders. The use of brand names, product names, common names, trade names, product descriptions etc. even without a particular marking in this work is in no way to be construed to mean that such names may be regarded as unrestricted in respect of trademark and brand protection legislation and could thus be used by anyone.

Cover image: www.ingimage.com

This book is a translation from the original published under ISBN 978-620-2-80870-5.

Publisher:
Sciencia Scripts
is a trademark of
Dodo Books Indian Ocean Ltd., member of the OmniScriptum S.R.L Publishing group
str. A.Russo 15, of. 61, Chisinau-2068, Republic of Moldova Europe
Printed at: see last page
ISBN: 978-620-3-59506-2

CHRONIC OBSTRUCTIVE PULMONARY DISEASE:
ANATOMOCLINICAL APPROACH
AND ITS PULMONARY INVOLVEMENT
SUMMARY

Chronic obstructive pulmonary disease (COPD) is a respiratory disease characterised by airflow obstruction, generally progressive and associated with a chronic inflammatory process. It is a pathology on the rise worldwide and is mainly attributed to smoking and environmental pollution. Dyspnoea, cough and phlegm production are the most frequent symptoms in COPD and may precede spirometric changes for years. Dyspnea on effort, chronic and progressive, is the most characteristic symptom of the disease and its perception is variable, in which many patients do not mention it or find the reduction of respiratory capacity natural with age. Although it is considered an avoidable and treatable disease, with slow pulmonary deterioration, it is essential to understand its pathophysiology in order to control not only the symptoms, but also its risk factors, especially smoking. The present study was carried out as an integrative review of qualitative literature on COPD. To this end, a bibliographical survey was conducted between January and February 2021, using the following databases: Virtual Health Library (VHL), Medline and United States National Library of Medicine (USNLM).

Keywords: Chronic obstructive pulmonary disease; treatment; epidemiology.

ABSTRACT

Chronic obstructive pulmonary disease (COPD) is a respiratory disease characterized by airflow obstruction, usually progressive and associated with a chronic inflammatory process. It is a condition on the rise in the world, being attributed mainly to smoking and environmental pollution. Dyspnea, cough, and phlegm production are the most frequent symptoms in COPD and may precede spirometric changes for years. Chronic and progressive dyspnea on stress is the most characteristic symptom of the disease and its perception is variable, in which many patients do not report it or think it is natural to reduce respiratory capacity over the years. Although it is considered a preventable and treatable disease with slow pulmonary deterioration, it is essential to understand its pathophysiology to control not only symptoms, but also their risk factors, especially smoking. The present study was carried out in the form of an integrative review of the qualitative literature on the theme OF COPD. For this, a bibliographic survey was carried out between January and February 2021, using the following databases: Virtual Health Library (VHL), Medline and United States National Library of Medicine (USNLM).

Keywords: Chronic obstructive pulmonary disease; treatment; epidemiology.

INTRODUCTION

Exposure to noxious gases and particles, such as those derived from tobacco, provokes an inflammatory response in the lungs which, when exacerbated, will cause structural alterations. In the long term this inflammatory process culminates in the narrowing of the small airways and destruction of the lung parenchyma. These changes will cause a reduction in the elastic traction that keeps the distal airways open, causing their early closure, mainly during expiration and resulting in obstruction to the airflow, giving characteristics to the disease called chronic obstructive pulmonary disease (COPD) (LOIVOS, 2019).

The main symptoms of COPD are dyspnoea, cough (often chronic), expectoration, wheezing and chest tightness. Chronic inflammation may generate chronic bronchitis, obstructive bronchiolitis and pulmonary emphysema, as well as important systemic alterations. Associated with the patient's clinical history, spirometry is a test that can lead to the diagnosis of COPD. Poorly controlled asthma can mimic COPD, that is, usually the symptoms of the two chronic inflammations are differentiated, but may remain similar in certain individuals, making the differential diagnosis difficult (SPANISH, 2010).

The WHO considers that 65 million people worldwide have moderate to severe COPD and project that by 2020, it will be the third leading cause of mortality. In addition, COPD is one of the leading causes of morbidity worldwide. In Brazil, the prevalence of COPD is estimated at 7.3 million individuals (AZAMBUJA et al., 2013).

According to data from the Brazilian Ministry of Health, COPD costs the public coffers approximately R$ 100 million annually, and about 70% of the patients depend on SUS for treatment. Considering the high incidence of respiratory diseases in the Brazilian population, the development of low-cost techniques for diagnosis and follow-up of these patients would result in significant economy of resources. The treatment for COPD is based on the degree of severity of the disease, which is classified according to diagnosis. Spirometry, together with chest X-ray and clinical evaluation of the patient, constitute the means of classification (ALVES, 2014).

Advanced age, loss of lung function and the stage of the disease before admission are important risk factors for increased mortality in these hospitalized patients. In addition, exacerbations have a serious negative impact on patients' quality of life and subsequent lung function, as well as on socioeconomic costs (MARCHIORI, et al., 2010).

Some patients have resistance to treatment, and education shows favorable results in treatment adherence, especially in elderly patients. It is important to understand how public policies, educational assistance to professionals and the understanding of the patients' needs are essential for the diagnosis and treatment of chronic obstructive pulmonary disease to be efficient and promote quality of life for patients (POSADA, 2011).

CHAPTER 1 - CONCEPTUAL APPROACHES TO ANATOMY AND RESPIRATORY PHYSIOLOGY

1.1 Morphofunctional analysis of the lungs

The lungs are the vital organs of respiration. Its main function is to oxygenate the blood by placing the inspired air very close to the venous blood in the pulmonary capillaries (MOORE and DALEY, 2014). The functional plan of the thorax facilitates this complex process. By acting together, the muscles of breathing and the diaphragm increase the intrathoracic volume, create a negative pressure in the pleural space surrounding the lung and cause the latter to expand. The consequent reduction of intra-alveolar pressure leads to the conduction of air through the upper respiratory tract to the trachea and airways and from there to the alveoli, in which gas exchange occurs (GRAYS, 2010).

Each lung is covered by the pleura, a serous membrane arranged like a closed invaginated sac. The visceral or pulmonary pleura adheres closely to the lung surface and its interlobar fissures. Its continuation, the parietal pleura, lines the corresponding half of the chest wall and covers much of the diaphragm and structures occupying the mid-thoracic region. The visceral and parietal pleurae are continuous with each other around the hilar structures and remain in intimate contact, though sliding over each other, in all phases of breathing. The parietal and visceral pleurae develop from the somatopleural and splancnopleural layers of the lateral plate mesoderm, respectively, which means that the parietal pleura is supplied by arteries from somatic sources. The visceral pleura constitutes an integral part of the lung and, therefore, its arterial supply and venous drainage are provided by the bronchial vessels (GRAYS, 2010).

Each lung has an apex, a base, three edges and two surfaces. In shape each lung approximates to half of a cone. The apex, the rounded upper end, protrudes above the thoracic aperture, where it makes contact with the cervical pleura and is covered in turn by the suprapleural membrane. The basal surface is semilunar and concave and rests on the upper surface of the diaphragm, which separates the right lung from the right lobe of the liver and the left lung from the left lobe of the liver, gastric fundus and spleen (GRAYS, 2010).

The right lung presents right oblique and horizontal fissures, which divide it into three right lobes: upper, middle and lower. The right lung is larger and heavier than the left, however it is shorter and wider, because the right dome of the diaphragm is higher and the heart and pericardium are more turned to the left. The anterior margin of the right lung is relatively straight. The left lung has a single left oblique fissure, which divides it into two left lobes, upper and lower. The anterior margin of the left lung has a deep cardiac incisure, an impression left by the deviation of the apex of the heart to the left side (MOORE and DALEY, 2014).

The lungs are attached to the mediastinum by the roots of the lungs - that is, the bronchi (and associated bronchial vessels), pulmonary arteries, superior and inferior pulmonary veins, pulmonary nerve plexuses (sympathetic, parasympathetic and visceral afferent fibres) and lymphatic vessels. From the larynx, the walls of the airways are supported by horseshoe or C-shaped rings of hyaline cartilage. The sub-laryngeal airways form the tracheobronchial tree. The trachea situated in the superior mediastinum is the trunk of the tree. It bifurcates at the level of the transverse plane of the thorax (or angle of the sternum) into main bronchi, one for each lung, which follow in an inferolateral direction and enter the hilum of the lungs. The right main bronchus is wider, shorter and more vertical than the left main bronchus because it enters directly into the hilum of the lung The left main bronchus follows inferolaterally, inferiorly to the aortic arch and anteriorly to the oesophagus and the thoracic part of the aorta, to reach the hilum of the lung. In the lungs, the bronchi branch constantly and give rise to the tracheobronchial tree. Each main (primary) bronchus divides into secondary lobar bronchi, two on the left and three on the right, each of which supplies a lobe of the lung. Each lobar bronchus divides into several tertiary segmental bronchi, which supply the bronchopulmonary segments. (MOORE and DALEY, 2014).

In addition to the tertiary segmental bronchi, there are 20 to 25 generations of branched conducting bronchioles that end as terminal bronchioles, the smallest conducting bronchioles. The wall of the bronchioles has no cartilage. The conducting bronchioles carry air, but have no glands or alveoli. Each terminal bronchiole gives rise to several generations of respiratory bronchioles, characterised by thin-walled, scattered pockets (alveoli) that originate from their lights. The pulmonary alveolus is the basic structural unit of gas exchange in the lung. Thanks to the presence of the alveoli, the respiratory bronchioles participate in both air transport and gas exchange. Each respiratory bronchiole gives rise to 2 to 11 alveolar ducts, and each of these gives rise to 5 to 6 alveolar sacs. The alveolar ducts are elongated airways, densely lined by alveoli, which lead to common spaces, the alveolar sacs, in which groups of alveoli open. New alveoli continue to develop until about 8 years of age, at which time there are approximately 300 million alveoli. (MOORE and DALEY, 2014).

The rate of alveolar ventilation is regulated by the nervous system to maintain the oxygen tension in arterial blood (partial pressure of oxygen [Po2]) and the carbon dioxide tension (carbon dioxide pressure [PCo2]) at relatively constant levels under a variety of conditions. Respiratory centres are composed of three main groups of neurons: *the dorsal respiratory group* generates inspiratory action potentials in a constantly increasing state and is responsible for the basic rhythm of breathing; the *pneumotaxic centre,* located dorsally in the upper part of the pons, helps control the rate and pattern of breathing by transmitting inhibitory signals to the dorsal respiratory group and thus controls the expansion phase of the respiratory cycle; the *ventral respiratory group,* located in the ventrolateral part of the medulla, can cause expiration or inspiration, depending on which neurons in the group are stimulated. The ventral respiratory group is inactive during normal quiet breathing, but stimulates the abdominal expiratory muscles when higher levels of breathing are required (GUYTON, 2017).

Respiratory muscles are morphologically and functionally skeletal muscles. The skeletal muscles, microscopically, are made up of muscle fibers composed of structures called myofibrils and their subunits constitute the functional unit of skeletal muscle known as sarcomere. The myofibrils are the contractile elements of the muscle. Each myofibril contains protein filaments: thin filament (actin) and thick filament (myosin). The thin filament is anchored in a firm transverse band (Z-line) and the gap between two Z-lines delimits the sarcomere. The myosin filaments are stabilized longitudinally by a protein called titin. This protein is extremely elastic. It helps to keep the myosin filaments in the centre of the sarcomere, ensures homogeneous force production and is involved in passive force generation at the level of the sarcomere (DUMKE, 2012).

Muscle fibres have anatomo-functional differences that aim to optimise muscle performance under different conditions and demands. The slow fibres with high oxidative potential (type I) are especially suitable for prolonged aerobic activities and are more resistant to fatigue. The fast fibers (type II) have higher glycolytic potential, are more susceptible to fatigue and less efficient in the use of O_2, which makes them useful in anaerobic exercise of high intensity and short duration (DUMKE, 2012).

The inspiratory muscle group includes the diaphragm, the external intercostals, the scalenes (SCS) and the sternocleidomastoid (SCM). The diaphragm is the main muscle of inspiration. During contraction of the diaphragm, the muscle fibres generate a caudal force on the central tendon in order to expand the thoracic cavity along its craniocaudal axis. The ECM and ESC muscles are considered accessory muscles of inspiration (DUMKE, 2012). The physiological action of the diaphragm is the elevation of the last six pairs of ribs, both laterally and anteriorly, and its anterior bundles elevate the sternum, increasing the transverse and anteroposterior diameter (LIMA and SANTANA, 2011).

Thus, its mobile point is in the thoracic periphery and its fixed point is constituted by a central fibrous tendon in contact with the spine. Only the diaphragm acts in small and medium amplitude inspiration, acting mainly on the lower lobes. In the inspiration of great amplitude, besides this muscle, the other inspiratory muscles elevate the upper ribs, promoting action on the lobes and upper bronchi. In forced expiration, the contraction of the expiratory muscles and the constrictive force of the lungs combine and predominate in relation to the passive force of the thorax and the airways close, expelling the air contained in the lungs, generating a high intrapleural pressure, displacing the tendinous centre of the diaphragm in a cranial direction. The expiratory muscles are: the transverse abdominis, the rectus abdominis and the internal and external obliques of the abdomen (LIMA e SANTANA, 2011).

1.2 Epidemiological indices

We can say that the world is experiencing a global epidemic of COPD. The WHO considers that: 1) 65 million people in the world have COPD of moderate to severe intensity; 2) more than 3 million COPD patients died in the year 2005; 3) in 2002, COPD was the fifth cause of mortality worldwide and 4) in 2020, it will be the third cause of mortality. In addition, COPD is one of the leading causes of morbidity worldwide. In Brazil, the prevalence of COPD is estimated at 7.3 million individuals. Since the smoking epidemic first affected males, mortality among males is still higher than among females.

Subsequently, there was an increase in the incidence of smoking among women, which justifies the rise of the COPD mortality curve in females (AZANBUJA, 2013).

In our country, there has been a progressive increase in the number of deaths from COPD in both sexes over the last 20 years. In 2011, the National Cancer Institute published that 15.1% of the population (190,732,694 million people) are smokers, which represents the main risk factor for COPD. It is known that approximately 15% of these develop COPD (AZANBUJA, 2013).

Considering the data from the 2010 Census, the Brazilian elderly population was accounted for 20,590,599 people. Analyzing the hospitalizations per age group, it was observed that the most affected group, in the total reported, was the group that comprises the population aged between 70 and 79 years, with a total of 158,627 cases. According to IBGE data, the population comprised in this range was equivalent to 6,305,085 people, the second range with the largest number of individuals. The mean number of cases per year, according to the data analyzed, in individuals between 70 and 79 years of age was approximately 31,725 cases of hospitalization for COPD. Since the geographic data date from 2010, it is possible to have only a projection of the quantity relative to the total population of the region. It is noteworthy that COPD is more reported in the older population in the range above 75 years, where the effects of aging are more exacerbated and affect the structure, function and also the control of the respiratory system. The prevalence of the disease increases with age, being notably higher after 65 years of age (BELO, BATISTA, & JUNIOR, 2016).

In Brazil, COPD is the third cause of death among chronic noncommunicable diseases, with a 12% increase in the number of deaths between 2005 and 2010, which currently represents almost 40,000 annual deaths resulting from COPD. In addition, COPD was responsible for a per cost of 103 million reais to the Unified Health System in 2011, referring to 142,635 hospitalizations. This cost was higher than that of patients with acute myocardial infarction and hypertension and was equivalent to that of patients with diabetes. According to the National Coordination of Tobacco Control and Primary Cancer Prevention of the National Cancer Institute, between 85% and 90% of all deaths from COPD are attributable to smoking (RABAHI, 2013).

Figure 1 - Number of hospitalizations in the Unified Health System for COPD and other chronic noncommunicable diseases in Brazil in 2011.

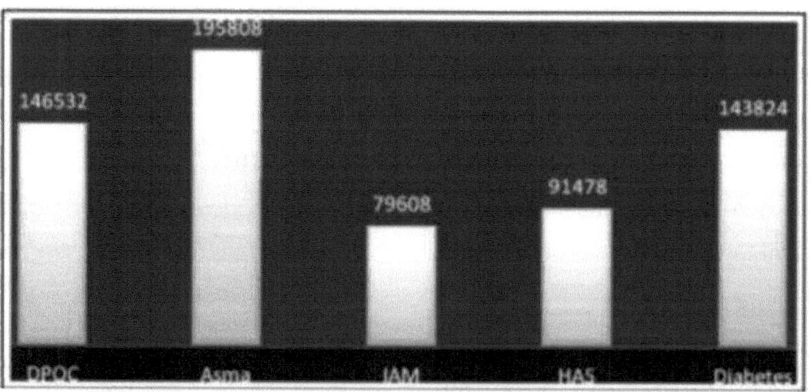

Source: Rabahi, 2013.

The region with the lowest number of ICD-10 notifications related to COPD was the Northern region. The North region is the second least populated region in Brazil, with approximately 15,864,454 inhabitants and an elderly population of 1,081,469 people. Only 19,308 cases of hospitalizations for COPD were reported in this region between 2012 and 2016, corresponding to 1.8% of the elderly population. This fact raises questions about the quality and access to health services in the North region, to the mortality rates and motivates questions about these low rates, which is not the object of this study. It is interesting to note that the Southeast region, even being the most populous, was not the region with the highest prevalence, being the second ranked, with 149,343 hospitalizations (BELO, BATISTA e JUNIOR, 2016).

In Brazil, 1,482,813 deaths were registered in the elderly population from 2012 to 2016, according to the SUS Hospital Information System. The number of deaths registered in the SIH/SUS having as cause the ICD-10 referring to COPD, in the population aged 60 years or more, was 36,687. The region with the highest number of deaths, taking into account all ICD-10 categories, was the Southeast, which has the largest number of elderly population, 9,527,354 individuals. This allows correlating the demographic data with the number of deaths, in addition, the greater exposure to risk factors by the inhabitants of this Brazilian region (BELO, BATISTA and JUNIOR, 2016).

Exposure to tobacco is the principal etiology of the disease, but other environmental pollutants, such as particles and gases (biomass burning), are also important and are amplified by factors that affect lung growth during pregnancy and childhood. However, other factors have also been implicated in the genesis of COPD, since only 15-20% of smokers develop the symptoms of the disease. Exposure to biomass has been one such factor that has been the subject of numerous publications; worldwide, nearly 3 billion people are exposed to smoke from biomass combustion, either for cooking or as an energy source for domestic heating. In these places, including a large part of the rural population in Brazil, domestic pollution is also responsible for the etiology of COPD. In a study conducted in Brazil evaluating 160 women recruited in basic health units who had a mean cumulative exposure to wood smoke of 211.2 ± 98.2 hours-year, 47 (29.4%) were diagnosed with COPD (RABAHI, 2013).

In this way, considering the current health conditions of the population, with the increase in life expectancy, the recent investigation of new determinants of COPD and evaluations of impact on the use of health services (including costs of care) should contribute to a better understanding of COPD and, consequently, provide subsidies for the control of this disease (RABAHI, 2013).

1.3 Risk factors

Smoking is the main risk factor for COPD. Approximately 1 in 5 smokers will develop the disease. In nonsmokers, the ratio is extremely low, 1 in 20 nonsmokers (~4%). Thus, active and passive smoking is directly related to the inflammatory process and the development of airflow limitation, with low reversibility to the use of bronchodilator drugs (RUFINO, COSTA, 2013). The risk of developing COPD in smokers is related to the dose, age of onset of the habit and total packs consumed, factors that are also related to mortality from the disease. Despite the above, COPD is "underdiagnosed" since only 15 to 20% of smokers are diagnosed with COPD, even though most of them develop airflow obstruction (LOIVOS, 2019).

Fetal exposure to smoking during pregnancy is the most important and potentially preventable assault on lung growth and development and may be associated with sudden infant death, intrauterine growth restriction, low birth weight and prematurity30. All these events have the potential to increase the risk of progression to an outcome of poorer lung function in early adulthood, and consequently increased risk for COPD (TONIDANDEL, 2019).

COPD is a polygenic disease and a classic example of gene-environment interaction. The best documented risk factor is marked deficiency of alpha-1- antitrypsin, the main inhibitor of serum proteases. It is a rare recessive trait, characterized by the early development of pan-lobular emphysema, and may be present in non-smoking patients, however being more common in smokers, evidencing the interaction between genetic predisposition and exposure to external factors - mainly smoking (LOIVOS, 2019).

Dust and chemical substances presented by occupational exposure (such as vapours, particles and fumes) stand out in this group of risk factors, which can demonstrably cause or increase the risk of developing COPD when there is prolonged contact with these elements (LOIVOS, 2019). Despite technological advances in the energy supply sectors, approximately 50% of the world's population and 90% of homes located in rural areas use the burning of biomass fuels in the form of wood, coal, animal dung or crop product waste, which produces high rates of air pollution, especially indoors. This suggests that smoke inhalation from the incomplete burning of these forms of fuel would be the main global risk factor for the development of COPD (TONIDANDEL, 2019).

Infections play an important role in the development of COPD. On the one hand, infections in young people predispose the individual to bronchiectasis or alterations in the airway response; on the other, COPD exacerbations are related to viral or bacterial infections. HIV infection has been shown to accelerate the onset of tobacco-related emphysema and tuberculosis constitutes, in addition to a differential diagnosis and potential comorbidity, a risk factor (GIL, FREITAS, & CORDEIRO, 2013).

An association between mucus hypersecretion and decline in VEMS (Maximal Expiratory Volume in the first second) has been found and, in young adult smokers, the presence of chronic bronchitis is associated with greater susceptibility to develop COPD (GIL, FREITAS and CORDEIRO, 2013).

1.4 Etiopathogenesis and pathophysiology of COPD

As regards its etiopathogenesis, Araújo and Drummond, as cited by Bugalho (2016), state that in COPD, the persistent inhalation of particles or noxious gases leads to anatomopathological changes that occur predominantly in the airways, but also in the lung parenchyma and muscles. Thus, chronic inflammation occurs in the airways, with hyperplasia of the mucoid glands, fibrosis and obstruction of the small airways. Regarding the pulmonary parenchyma, a destruction of the structures distal to the terminal bronchiole may be observed, resulting in the presence of emphysema. Hyperplasia of the intima and smooth muscle occurs in the pulmonary vessels and in the context of chronic vasoconstriction secondary to hypoxia (FERNANDES, 2019).

Apparently all smokers have large airway injury, but only a variable percentage of them also have airway injury with a diameter of 2 mm or less. COPD patients, therefore, have both large and small airway mucosal lesions, which are sequential or nearly simultaneous, but certainly happen first in the proximal airways. The circumstances which allow in some of the smokers that the action of toxic gases and fumes extends to the small-calibre airways, as noted above, must be many. However, one may speculate that variations in the structure of the bronchial tree may collaborate to the development of COPD. A simplification in the branching pattern of the bronchial tree, whether resulting from failure in the process of bronchial generation during gestation or else acquired in the postnatal period, as a result of infection, may facilitate the entry of toxic substances in peripheral areas of the lung, which would be more protected if the complex branching of the bronchioles forced these gases and particles to travel tortuous paths (PASCHOAL and MOREIRA, 2016).

It is also important to mention that besides a pulmonary component, COPD has an extrapulmonary component, which contributes to the severity of the disease. The clinical picture and the repercussions of the person's general health status are influenced by the systemic manifestations of COPD, and it is often associated with other diseases/ disorders, namely cardiovascular diseases, metabolic syndrome, osteoporosis, weight loss, musculoskeletal dysfunction, depression and lung cancer (FERNANDES, 2019).

It is now known that under some circumstances, such as infection and smoking, inflammatory cells, especially leukocytes and macrophages, migrate in large numbers to the lung. There, they are activated and generate an inflammatory reaction which, over the years, has consequences on the structure and functionality of the lungs. This inflammatory process occurs in the small airways (< 2 mm), being normally tenuous and continuous, originating the coalescence of alveoli and alveolar ducts in an irregular and definitive way (RUFINO and COSTA, 2013).

The inflammatory cells that are recruited in COPD release substances such as elastase, collagenases and oxidant products, which, superimposed on the oxidants inhaled from cigarette smoke, act by modifying the components of the extracellular matrix. Thus, the lung acquires a new, deformed model (stretching and disappearance of the alveolar tabs forming larger air spaces and bronchial compressions associated with areas of hyperinflation), irreversible and leading to the impairment of one of the most primitive functions of life, which is the very act of breathing. In histopathological studies of patients with COPD, using immunohistochemical methods, the CD8+ T lymphocyte count is significantly higher than in control groups. The lymphocyte participation in COPD was the main and most recent advance in its pathogenesis (RUFINO, COSTA, 2013).

Saetta et al., (1998), refer that the principal inflammatory cells that mediate inflammation in COPD are macrophages, dendritic cells, neutrophils, eosinophils and cytotoxic TCD8+ lymphocytes. These inflammatory cells present in the submucosa of the airways of COPD patients are enlarged and some of them stimulate the release of proteases (enzymes that destroy cell membrane proteins) and oxidants that damage the extracellular matrix of the lungs, disrupt normal lung repair mechanisms, inactivate alpha-1-antitrypsin and promote apoptosis or senescence of extracellular matrix-producing lung cells. Although the presence of eosinophils is a characteristic of asthma, in COPD exacerbation there may be an increase in the number of these cells mediated by an increase in cytokines, responsible for the migration of eosinophils and the inflammatory response (TANDO, 2016).

Oxidative stress may be an important amplifying mechanism in COPD. Oxidative stress biomarkers (e.g. hydrogen peroxide, 8-isoprostane) are increased in exhaled and condensed air, mucus and systemic circulation of COPD patients. Oxidative stress is more increased in exacerbations. Oxidants originate from cigarette smoke and other inhaled particles, and are released from activated inflammatory cells such as macrophages and neutrophils. A reduction in endogenous antioxidants may also occur in COPD patients. Oxidative stress has several adverse consequences in the lungs, including activation of inflammatory genes, inactivation of antiproteases, stimulation of mucus secretion, and stimulation of increased plasma esxudation (SPANHOL, 2011).

From the pathophysiological point of view, COPD is characterised by airway inflammation caused by exposure to risk factors, such as inhaled dust and gases and tobacco, which leads to the narrowing of the small airways and the destruction of the parenchyma, with loss of alveolar connections and decreased lung elastic retraction. These changes lead to an increase in expiratory time and residual volume with consequent lung hyperinflation (ROCHA, 2017).

Figure 2 - Characterization of COPD from the pathophysiological point of view

Pathophysiology of COPD	Mucous hypersecretion	- ciliated epithelial cell metaplasia - chronic productive cough
	Airway remodelling	- narrowing and fibrosis of the airways - increased small airway resistance - reduction in the calibre of the bronchi - loss of elastic retraction force due to parenchymal destruction
	Limitation of air debts	- reduction in FEV, - reduction in the FEVi/ FVC ratio - static hyperinflation due to decreased inspiratory capacity at tidal volume (due to increased residual volume) - dynamic hyperinflation due to increased functional residual capacity
	Limitation of respiratory muscles	- mechanical disadvantage of the diaphragm - muscle atrophy may occur

	Changes in the ventilation-perfusion relation	- heterogeneity of ventilation due to destruction of alveolar units - heterogeneity of perfusion distribution due to destruction of alveolar capillaries - changes in gas exchange with hypoxaemia and hypercapnia - changes in carbon monoxide diffusion
	Cor pulmonale	- increased pressure in the pulmonary circulation - pulmonary hypertension - right ventricular hypertrophy - right-sided heart failure

Source: Rocha, 2017.

The decreased retractable capacity of the lung and the blockage of the thorax in the inspiratory position result from the obstruction of the airways and cause the horizontalisation of the costal arches, creating a straightening and depression of the diaphragm, as well as the consequent shortening of the inspiratory muscles. This aspect translates into superior costal breathing with recourse to the accessory muscles of breathing and inspiratory retraction of the lower ribs and abdomen. These alterations in the respiratory process lead to an increase in respiratory work, dyspnoea, muscular fatigue and hypoxia. Mucous hypersecretion may also be observed as a result of mucous metaplasia, this increase being produced by the submucosal glands in response to the inflammatory process present. This hypersecretion of mucus may lead to a chronic cough. The progression of the disease promotes the compromising of gas exchange, generates hypoxemia and hypercapnia and originates abnormalities in the ventilation-perfusion relation with worsening of symptoms. The determination of the FEV1/FVC ratio after bronchodilation confirms the diagnosis of the disease (ROCHA, 2017).

1.5 Systemic effects of COPD

It is recognised that COPD may be associated with several comorbidities, with high impact on quality of life. The alterations resulting from the pathophysiological process of the disease may lead to the presence of systemic effects. Alteration in heart function is one of these systemic effects, resulting from airflow limitation and pulmonary hyperinflation. Others may be named, such as myopathy and/or muscle atrophy, cachexia/malnutrition and may even initiate or worsen comorbidities such as osteoporosis, anaemia, diabetes, metabolic syndromes and depression. Inflammatory mediators are thought to be primarily responsible for the onset of these changes. Another systemic effect of COPD is skeletal muscle dysfunction, which results from muscle depelation (FERREIRA, 2014).

Respiratory muscles, particularly the diaphragm, start to have their fibers shortened due to pulmonary hyperinflation, leading to functional muscle weakness. Diaphragmatic adaptive changes include: 1) the ability to generate higher transdiaphragmatic pressure than healthy individuals during non-volitional contraction at equivalent high lung volumes; 2) diaphragm sarcomere length is shorter according to the degree of lung hyperinflation; 3) cellular adaptations in response to hyperinflation, including an increase in the concentration of mitochondria in muscle cells and changes in the types and configurations of myofibres recruited during respiration. In addition to the diaphragm, there are several similar adaptive changes reported in other respiratory muscles, for example, the external intercostals. Despite these impressive temporal adaptations, the presence of severe lung hyperinflation and reduced inspiratory capacity means that the ventilatory reserve in COPD is diminished and the ability to increase ventilation when demand increases suddenly, as in exercise or exacerbation, is very limited (VIEIRA, 2017).

The scientific evidence supports the role of physical inactivity as a major factor in the development of musculoskeletal dysfunction in the person with COPD. According to some authors (Kim et al, 2008; Marquis et al, 2002), this systemic effect predicts mortality more effectively than pulmonary function status. However, the changes resulting from the pathophysiological process of the disease and the factors associated with its development are also pointed out as reasons for skeletal muscle dysfunction (FERREIRA, 2014).

Individuals with COPD may also experience difficulty in upper limb exercise. This difficulty is partly due to changes in respiratory mechanics associated with the disease, so that muscles required for upper limb activities are also required for breathing. Consequently, when performing activities using their upper limbs, people with COPD may experience shortness of breath and early cessation of the task. Given that most activities of daily living require the use of the arms, breathlessness and early cessation of upper limb activities represent a challenge for people with COPD (VIEIRA, 2017).

Muscle dysfunction affects the way people with COPD experience their lives and develop their autonomy, thus being a very important focus of the rehabilitation process and of the rehabilitation nurse. Studies on this topic showed that inspiratory muscle strength was more affected than peripheral muscle strength (FERREIRA, 2014).

Various scientific evidences have confirmed the appearance of muscular dysfunctions in COPD patients. Among them, the following stand out: the attenuation of type I fibers; an atrophy of type I and II fibers; the modified levels of metabolic enzymes and the decreased capillarity. They also found that the isometric strength of the quadriceps muscles and respiratory muscles of individuals with COPD was reduced, as well as the ventilatory fitness of these individuals, which consequently contributed to the reduced tolerance to physical exercise (SANTOS, SENA, & COSTA, 2019). According to Simpson et al. the most evident worsening in exercise capacity was found in individuals with very severe obstruction, in addition to the greatest reduction in skeletal muscle strength indices. In the same study, there was a 33% increase in 1 RM of the upper limb exercise, comparing pre- and post-training. Ortega et al. also performed upper and lower limb strength training in individuals with COPD with moderate to severe obstruction, and found an increase in muscle strength in all exercises performed after treatment (IKE, et al., 2010).

Although COPD affects mainly the lungs, several extrapulmonary manifestations have been described, among them, the change in postural balance. Previous studies in the literature have demonstrated significant balance deficits in the COPD population as compared with healthy individuals, with COPD patients showing damage in balance reactions in response to externally applied disturbances, which has a particular relevance in the risk of falling. Initially, Butcher et al. in 2004 compared COPD patients on or off supplemental oxygen with healthy individuals and the authors found that COPD patients showed deficits in functional balance, coordination and mobility associated with disease severity, but not associated with the use of supplemental oxygen. On the other hand, from evaluations carried out by Beauchamp et al. in 2009, it was found that balance damage and occurrence of falls commonly observed in COPD patients were associated with the use of supplemental oxygen. The authors suggest that this probably occurs due to the greater sedentary lifestyle of this group of patients and due to reduced motor coordination resulting from cerebral hypoxemia (PEREIRA, 2017).

The proprioceptive alteration that occurs in COPD patients and its relation with inspiratory muscle weakness has been the object of study as another possible factor associated with postural balance alterations in these patients. The study by Janssens et al. points out that COPD patients, especially those with inspiratory muscle weakness, have greater confidence on ankle proprioceptive signals and less confidence on dorsal proprioceptive signals, suggesting that inspiratory muscle weakness contributes to impaired proprioceptive postural control. Rocco et al. in 2011 demonstrated that patients with COPD of moderate to severe severity, compared to healthy individuals, in addition to balance and gait deficits, lower peripheral muscle strength and lower level of functional capacity, also showed reduced reflex response. These results suggest that, in addition to functional changes, COPD patients have neurophysiological impairments, such as changes in nerve conduction (PEREIRA, 2017).

There is increasing evidence that COPD is more than a physical disease, often accompanied by significant psychological and behavioural problems. From the psychological point of view, the disease brings with it a set of characteristics that reflect the most profound consequences at the levels of emotional, affective and relational balance. According to some authors, COPD patients have a rigid emotional and mental control, which allows the individual to avoid some conflicts, but may also generate others. When studying the psychological characteristics of COPD patients, Hynninem and colleagues (2005, apud SILVA et al., 2006) found a high level of social isolation, as well as feelings of ineffectiveness, insecurity and inferiority. There are patients who abandon activities that give meaning to their lives, and change to less demanding activities that also satisfy them. Others abandon and give up these activities completely, with feelings of impotence, isolation and uselessness. The functional limitations of the disease can lead the individual, to a temporary abstention from their job thus affecting their professional function and, consequently, their economic life (FARIAS, 2011).

Some studies suggest that patients with COPD may present decreased swallowing strength, use of exhaled air to clean the pharyngeal recesses, as well as desensitization of the larynx, which may increase the chance of penetration episodes and silent aspiration. Such factors may trigger aspiration pneumonias and disease exacerbation. In the study of Bassi et al. (2014), it was identified that COPD patients admitted to a university hospital were at risk for oropharyngeal dysphagia, ratifying the relationship between individuals with COPD and dysphagia symptoms. For these individuals, coordination between breathing and swallowing is very important, since episodes of tracheal aspiration resulting from swallowing disorders can lead to disease exacerbation. Conversely, an exacerbation of respiratory disease can lead to aspiration episodes, thus increasing the severity of the condition (PRESTES, et al., 2019).

Oropharyngeal dysphagia is a symptom that can cause bronchoaspiration and worsening of the respiratory condition. When the patient already has COPD and is diagnosed with oropharyngeal dysphagia, he or she has a higher risk of pulmonary complications because he or she may bronchospasm saliva, secretion, or food into a lung restricted by the obstructive disease. For these reasons, dysphagia should be diagnosed as early as possible and be assessed by a specialist so that techniques and strategies for safe swallowing are implemented, as well as better feeding conditions for the patient (ROSA, 2013).

According to Petty (2006), many COPD patients have an important psychological component characterised by anxiety and depression. The high prevalence of anxiety has been related to an emotional response to respiratory symptoms, being responsible for worsening dyspnoea and the whole clinical picture, often leading the patient to be hospitalised. For the same author, this may be the reason why nicotine dependence is so powerful in COPD patients. Nicotine helps to alleviate these uncomfortable symptoms and perceptions (FARIAS, 2011).

Advanced age is associated with worse quality of life scores, causing greater impact by impairing activities of daily living and work. When two or more factors are associated, this impact seems to be even greater. The quality of life of the elderly has often been associated with dependency-autonomy issues; dependency results from biological changes and consequently from social changes. In a study describing the factors associated with the degree of satisfaction with life in an elderly population, the authors emphasise that health and independence are the main determinants of a better quality of life. Other factors mentioned were: support system, being accepted by the community, affectivity, positive description of marriage and family conditions that reinforce the perception of social and family life (KERKOSKI, BORESTEIN, & SILVA, 2010).

Depressive disorder and suicide are related to smoking habit, the leading cause of COPD. It was also noted in the study by Clyde et al (2013) that smoking habit is associated with depression. As well as people with depressive disorder feel stimulated to smoke. After diagnosis, people with COPD are advised and encouraged to quit smoking to reduce the progression of the disease. The nicotine present in tobacco is a psychoactive substance acting on the dopaminergic receptors in the nucleus accumbens and in the corpus striatum. The stimulation of dopaminergic receptors causes various behaviors such as: improvement in attention and memory, anxiety control, increased self-esteem and self-confidence, and modulation of mood. Considering the need to quit smoking and the association between nicotine dependence and depression, the withdrawal syndrome may present depressive symptoms when smoking is discontinued. Because most patients with COPD have some symptoms of anxiety or depression, they may represent a risk group for suicide (SAMPAIO, 2019).

COPD promotes structural, physiological and psychological changes in the lives of its patients, causing significant morbidity and mortality in those who are affected by the disease. In addition to the impact on the lives of patients, it promotes changes in the lives of their families, not only by spending health resources, but also by the repercussions on the daily lives of patients, including their quality of life (VIEIRA, 2017).

1.6 Clinical picture and diagnosis

The clinical suspicion of COPD should be considered in every individual aged 40 years or older (30 or 35 years according to some ongoing studies, still without validation) with a history of exposure to risk factors for this disease (tobacco, biomass fuels, occupational vapours or dust, etc.), accompanied or not by respiratory symptoms of the disease, which are mainly dyspnoea on effort, chronic cough and phlegm production (ZONZIN, et al., 2017).

Dyspnoea, cough and phlegm production are the most frequent symptoms in COPD and may precede spirometric alterations by years. Dyspnea on effort, chronic and progressive, is the most characteristic symptom. Its perception is variable, many patients do not report it or find natural the reduction of respiratory capacity with age (especially in the elderly). They end up adapting to effort dyspnea, reducing physical activity, starting with non-essential leisure activities and progressing to include basic daily life activities. This reduction in physical activity leads to deconditioning, which in turn aggravates dyspnea (ZONZIN, et al., 2017).

Chronic cough is often the first symptom. Persistent or episodic, it generally predominates in the morning period, and may be unproductive or productive with mucoid expectoration. It is a condition many times not mentioned by the patient, due to a distortion in the patient's perception, who interprets it, not as a symptom of a disease that is being installed, but as a natural and expected reaction of his body due to the habit of smoking. The simple verification of cough by the doctor during the examination can already show its occurrence and be a starting point in the search for a diagnosis. The increase in volume and purulence of the expectoration are useful in the identification of exacerbation episodes of the disease. Wheezing and chest tightness may be present. Fatigue and weight loss suggest a higher degree of severity of the disease or the development of additional complications such as lung cancer (ZONZIN, et al., 2017).

According to GOLD (2013), the main obstructive disorders that make up COPD are: chronic bronchitis and emphysema: a) chronic bronchitis - consists of inflammation of the bronchi; "it is a functional disorder, clinically defined as productive cough of sputum, daily for three months a year, for at least two successive years." (STEVENS; LOWE, 1998, p. 172). A remarkable characteristic in the pathogenesis of chronic bronchitis is the constant irritation of the respiratory tract, caused mainly by the inhalation of cigarette smoke;

b) pulmonary emphysema - is characterized by the abnormal and permanent increase of the air spaces distal to the terminal bronchiole, accompanied by the destruction of its walls without the incidence of fibrosis (COTRAN; KUMAR, COLLINS, 2000, p. 635). When emphysema occurs, the lungs lose elasticity, given that the respiratory tissue is destroyed; the alveoli are compromised and there is a decreased ability to perform gas exchange (healthy alveoli are numerous, very small, spongy and elastic (ALVES, 2014).

In the initial phases, usually no alterations are identified in the physical examination. As the disease progresses, manifestations such as hypersonority to precussion, diffusely reduced thoracovocal fremitus, teleinspiratory fine rales may appear. Snoring and wheezing may also be noticed in some cases. Tachypnea, breathing with half-closed lips and use of accessory muscles may be present varying according to the degree of severity of the disease (ZONZIN, et al., 2017).

Figure 3 - COPD severity grades

COPD Severity Grades	
Graul/ Slight	the person coughs frequently, sometimes sputum; feels some shortness of breath when working or walking fast; often the person does not know he has the disease yet.
Grade2/ Moderate	The person has more coughing and wheezing; feels short of breath when doing strenuous work or walking faster; it is normal for the person at this stage to seek medical help.
Grade 3/Gravity	The symptoms worsen; the person coughs frequently and with sputum; there is great difficulty in breathing even during activities that do not require much effort.
Grade 4/ More Serious	The person's quality of life is greatly affected and worsening symptoms can put the person's life at risk.

Source: Cordeiro and Menoita, 2012.

In terms of COPD diagnosis, there is a consensus between the different NOCs regarding the clinical presentation of the patient, the risk factors involved in the development of the disease, particularly tobacco, and the importance of using spirometry in the diagnosis. Spirometry is a functional lung test that allows measuring the exhaled air volume over time and thus assessing the existence or not of airflow limitation (COSTA, 2010).

GOLD (2018) highlights the FEV1/FVC ratio, to define the presence of COPD, this being a fixed ratio, always less than 70%. Cordeiro and

Menoita (2012) citing Gulini (2006) added that the post-bronchodilator FEV1 always remains below 80%. The DGS (2016) emphasises the importance of FEV1, and this value should be assessed in all COPD patients, because it correlates with the patient's maximal capacity for physical activity and, therefore, disease severity (FERNANDES, 2019).

Radiological findings, in general, are late manifestations in the natural history of this disease and are not always associated with functional alterations. Hyperinflation is the most important finding, reflecting the loss of elastic traction of the lungs. The rectification or lowering of the diaphragm below the sixth anterior intercostal space at maximum inspiration; the increase in retrosternal airway space (greater than 3 cm); and the elongation and verticalization of the transverse diameter of the heart, at its greatest extent, less than 11.5 cm and remaining tapered even with right ventricular enlargement, are criteria for pulmonary hyperinflation (MACHADO, et al., 2013).

Figure 4 - Posteroanterior chest radiography demonstrating signs of pulmonary hyperinflation (left). Lateral chest radiography demonstrating increase in the anteroposterior chest diameter and flattening of the diaphragmatic dome (right).

Source: Machado, et al., 2013.

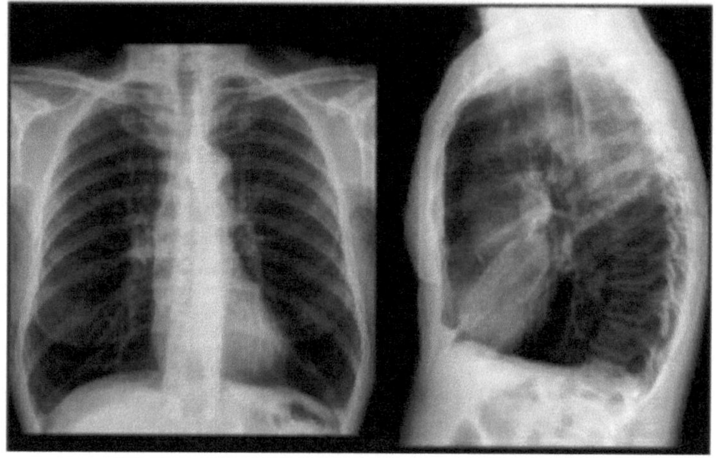

Chest computed tomography is only indicated in COPD in special cases, such as suspicion of the presence of bronchiectasis or bullae, indication for surgical correction or programming of volume reduction surgery. Pulse oximetry may initially be used for non-invasive oxygenation evaluation. If arterial oxygen saturation (SaO2) equal to or below 90% is identified, arterial gasometry (AG) is indicated (FERREIRA, 2010).

GA is an exam performed by collecting a blood sample from an artery, using a syringe and needle and the sample can be collected from the radial artery, the femoral artery or the brachial artery. After extraction, the blood is immediately sent to the laboratory for analysis (FERREIRA, 2010).

Finally, the diagnosis of COPD should be based on clinical symptoms, spirometry results and complementary tests (GA, X-rays, among others), but it should also take into account other important factors that influence the impact and evolution of this disease, such as: low body mass composition and decreased exercise capacity that are associated with high mortality risk, as well as decreased functional capacity (FERREIRA, 2010).

CHAPTER 2 - METHODOLOGICAL ASPECTS OF POCD

This study was conducted in the format of an integrative review of the qualitative type on the topic of Chronic Obstructive Pulmonary Disease (COPD). To this end, a bibliographical survey was conducted between January and February 2021, using the following databases: Virtual Health Library (VHL), PubMed and United States National Library of Medicine (USNLM). The following descriptors were used: chronic obstructive pulmonary disease, treatment, and epidemiology.

The inclusion criteria for the choice of articles included complete articles from the last eleven years (2009-2020), in Portuguese and English. The exclusion criteria were papers that, despite contemplating the descriptors of this study did not contain sufficient information about the subject researched.

CHAPTER 3 - PULMONARY CHANGES IN OPCD AND TREATMENTS

3.1 Pulmonary alterations in COPD

Generally, patients with COPD present weakness of the inspiratory muscles, which is associated with reduced performance of the diaphragm. This reduction in muscle strength can be explained, in part, by metabolic adaptations that occur in this musculature, where there is a predominance of slow fibers with high oxidative capacity (type I) and, as demonstrated by Stubbing et al., type I diaphragm fibers produce less strength when compared to type II fibers (DUMKE, 2012).

In patients with COPD, pulmonary resistance is increased due to the diffuse reduction of the bronchial lumen which causes relative obstruction of the airflow. Hypersecretion, oedema and spasm are factors responsible for bronchial obstruction and cause major alterations in respiratory dynamics. During the crisis, inspiration becomes rapid and superficial, while expiration increases its momentum and does not allow the efficient exit of air, causing pulmonary hyperinflation. Dyspnea is directly associated to tachypnea, as the patient tries to maintain the minute-volume in the face of severe obstruction in the expiratory phase. Functionally, lung hyperinflation is characterized by increased functional residual capacity that determines considerable change in respiratory muscle mechanics, compromising the ability of the ventilatory pump to sustain spontaneous breathing (LIMA and SANTANA, 2011).

The dynamic compliance of the respiratory system decreases

and the positive end-expiratory pressure (intrinsic PEEP) imposes an inspiratory load threshold that must be exceeded before inspiratory flow occurs. Total lung capacity may remain normal or slightly increased. Like all obstructive respiratory insufficiency the thorax is blocked in inspiration. As the crisis occurs, alterations in respiratory mechanics become more pronounced, for example, the lowering of the diaphragmatic hemispheres results in a lower abdominal pressure and, consequently, in a lower expansion of the lower thoracic cage leading to a decrease of costal mobility. This process causes shortening of the ventilatory muscles, generating a mechanical disadvantage to meet the needs of the respiratory demand. The chest blocked in inspiration results in an excessive and permanent tension of the musculoaponeurotic chains, being called chest in tonnage (LIMA and SANTANA, 2011).

Changes in the structural cells of the respiratory tract under the action of tobacco smoke may represent, in a simplistic view, the end result of aggression of the respiratory tract, reducing it to the cause-effect binomial, or introduce in this premise the complex interactions of biological dynamics, constituting, according to Puchelle, a form of self-protection and repair of tobacco-induced lesions. In the central airways, the epithelium's response to aggression is translated by the transformation of the ciliated cylindrical epithelium into squamous metaplasia, with impairment of mucociliary clearance and increased risk of developing carcinoma (MARQUES, 2014).

The damage caused by cigarettes in the lungs affects the airway epithelium and alveolar walls. Initially, the efficiency of the ciliary beat is impaired, then the cilia themselves are destroyed and finally the ciliated cell dies. Ciliated cells are differentiated cells that no longer have the ability to enter into mitosis. The loss of ciliated cells stimulates the secretory cells to divide. The persistence of the noxious stimulus (cigarette smoke) leads to a situation of excessive production of mucus and deficient transport (secretory metaplasia and decreased transport due to the lower number and activity of the cilia) (GONÇALVES, 2010).

For reasons as yet unidentified, most smokers manage to restrict the lesion produced by cigarette smoking to the epithelium of the large airways. In a fraction of this population of smokers, however, this lesion will extend to the small airways, located from the fifteenth generation of bronchi. In these circumstances, the secretion produced in these regions of the lung is retained and starts to function as a culture medium for bacteria which are no longer eliminated by the mucociliary apparatus. The aggression of the toxic products of cigarette smoke and the presence of bacteria trigger an inflammatory process

bronchiolar lumen which is temporally heterogeneous: there are bronchioles in the acute phase of inflammation, bronchioles in the subacute phase of the inflammatory process and bronchioles with lumen diminished by a fibrotic process which is the sequel of a chronic inflammation (GONÇALVES, 2010).

Smokers with COPD may present preponderant structural alterations in alveoli. The enlargement of the distal air spaces that results from the destruction of alveolar septa and from the transformation of various alveoli into single air spaces draws attention in these individuals. A large part of the pulmonary elasticity, responsible for passive expiration, independent of the action of expiratory muscles, is given by the elastic fibers that compose the alveolar septum. The progressive disappearance of many alveolar septa decreases pulmonary elasticity and, as a result, also decreases the elastic pressure that generates the expiratory flow. The increase in the air spaces distal to the terminal bronchiole with destruction of alveolar walls defines pulmonary emphysema (PASCHOAL and MOREIRA, 2016).

A recent histological evaluation of a large number of cases has shown that thickening of all layers of the small airway wall, filling of the lumen by mucus, and the intensity of the inflammatory response correlate with the progression of COPD, as assessed by FEV1. The reduced lumen of the bronchioles is also responsible for the onset of chronic respiratory failure in patients with chronic obstructive smoking bronchitis: the reduction of ventilation caused by bronchiolar stenosis allows the appearance of poorly ventilated areas with maintained perfusion, a fact that causes the oxygen concentration in the arterial blood to drop (GONÇALVES, 2010).

In most cases, the individual smoker, susceptible to the harmful effects of cigarettes, has both types of lesion, of the bronchioles and the alveolar septa. Therefore, chronic obstructive bronchitis and pulmonary emphysema coexist in the same patient with COPD. However, it is also possible, in most situations, to classify the patient as more markedly bronchitic or more emphysematous (GONÇALVES, 2010).

In the small airways squamous metaplasia appears not only to increase with disease severity, but also to contribute to peribronchiolar fibrosis through secretion of interleukin-1p and activation of fibroblasts, with increased Transforming Growth Factor (TGF-p) production, which amplifies pathological epithelio-mesenchymal transformation (MARQUES, 2014).

Pathological changes in the lungs lead to physiological changes characteristic of the disease, including mucus hypersecretion, ciliary dysfunction, respiratory flow limitation, pulmonary hyperdilatation, gas exchange abnormalities and pulmonary hypertension. They usually develop, in this order, as the disease progresses. Mucous hypersecretion and ciliary dysfunction lead to chronic cough and sputum production. These symptoms may be present for many years before other symptoms or physiological abnormalities develop. Limitation of respiratory flow, measured by spirometry, is the characteristic physiological change of COPD and the key to the diagnosis of the disease. It is mainly caused by fixed airway obstruction and the consequent increase in airway resistance. The destruction of alveolar connections, which inhibit the ability of the small airways to maintain permeability, plays a minor role (COSTA, 2014).

3.2 Therapeutic approach

The treatment of COPD aims to prevent disease progression, reduce symptoms, improve exercise tolerance, improve the patient's quality of life, and prevent acute exacerbations, thus reducing mortality. Patients in an advanced stage of the disease may undergo lung transplantation (TANDO, 2016).

The main measures for the management of stable COPD are: patient education, pharmacological and non-pharmacological treatment. Pharmacological therapy is used for prevention and control of symptoms, reduction of the frequency and severity of exacerbations, aiming at a general improvement in health status and increased quality of life (POSADA, 2011).

Figure 5 - Treatment of COPD (Adapted from Gold, 2016).

Non-pharmacological treatment	**Pharmacological treatment**
• Smoking Cessation • Physical activity • Pulmonary rehabilitation • Nutritional counselling • Ventilatory support Non-invasive ventilation Oxygen therapy • Surgical treatment	• Bronchodilatorcs • Agonists (fc adrenergic • Anticholinergics • Mctilxanthines • Combined bronchodilator therapy • Anti-inflammatories • Phosphodiesterase-4 inhibitors • Alpha substitution therapy 1 antitrypsin • Vaccination • Antibiotics

Source: TANDO, 2016.

Stopping smoking is the most important measure to be adopted by a patient with COPD. Orientation and inclusion in a smoking cessation support group can be decisive for the success of this therapy. The use of drugs to control nicotine abstention, such as bupropion or varenicline, can be an important aid in this regard. However, psychological support or cognitive behavioural therapy, especially when carried out in conjunction with nicotine replacement therapy or drug treatment, presents superior results. Rehabilitation is an important pillar in the treatment of COPD patients and should be thought of for all patients with any degree of disability. If the patient cannot be inserted in a respiratory rehabilitation programme, he/she should be encouraged to perform some type of physical activity. Patients with contraindications for physical exercise, such as unstable angina or recent infarction should be introduced into the program only after control of coronary disease (COSTA and RUFINO, 2013).

Although COPD is considered an obstructive disease of irreversible character, bronchodilators are the key elements in the treatment of the disease. The main classes of inhaled bronchodilators are anticholinergics and beta-2 agonists. Inhaled drugs are preferred over oral ones because they cause fewer side effects. 1,2 Every COPD patient with respiratory symptoms should be treated with bronchodilators, preferably long-acting or long-acting, as they reduce the frequency of exacerbations and hospitalisations, improve quality of life and reduce mortality. Anticholinergics act on the cholinergic system blocking the muscle constrictor effect on the bronchi. Ipratropium bromide is a short-acting anticholinergic that can be used in spray or nebulised form. Currently, it has been used as a rescue medication as long-acting bronchodilators are available. Tiotropium is the only long-acting anticholinergic and can be used in a single daily dose. Studies prove its superiority over placebo in the treatment of patients with stable COPD, with an increase in FEV1 in patients who used the drug (COSTA and RUFINO, 2013).

Beta-2 agonists cause bronchodilation by acting directly on bronchial muscle fibers. Thus, they are currently reserved for rescue, during worsening of dyspnea or in patients with mild disease who present dyspnea only after some exercise. Generally, two to four jets are prescribed up to every 4/4 hours, but patients requiring frequent doses of bronchodilators may be treated with long-acting or long-acting beta-2 agonists. Although they have an uncertain mechanism of action, xanthines have been used in the treatment of COPD for many years. With the development of inhaled drugs, xanthines have had their role restricted due to their side effects, especially epigastric pain and nausea, in addition to interaction with other drugs (COSTA and RUFINO, 2013).

Recently launched in Brazil, roflumilast is a nonsteroidal anti-inflammatory agent that inhibits phosphodiesterase 4, an enzyme that metabolises cyclic adenosine monophosphatase (cAMP) located in structural and inflammatory cells that participate in the COPD inflammatory process. It must be administered orally and interacts with cytochrome P450, being advisable not to associate it with theophylline and other drugs that act on this cytochrome. Although there is no large study on the use of supplemental oxygen in patients with COPD, it is accepted as an indication for oxygen therapy the presence of PaO2 < 55 mmHg, or between 56-59 mmHg in the presence of signs suggestive of cor pulmonale, congestive heart failure or erythrocytosis (hematocrit > 55%) (COSTA and RUFINO, 2013).

The Influenza vaccine reduces the onset of complications and mortality in 50% of patients and its repetition is indicated annually in autumn. The pneumococcal polysaccharide vaccine is recommended for patients over 65 years (POSADA, 2011).

Lung transplantation is an option for properly selected COPD patients with extremely advanced disease. It has proven to be a good option, improving the patient's functional capacity and quality of life.

(77-79) For this treatment the following criteria must be taken into consideration: FEV1 lower than 35% of predicted, PaO2 lower 7.3-8.0 kPa (55-60 mmHg), PaCO2 higher than 6.7 kPa (50 mm Hg), and secondary pulmonary hypertension. In addition to the above indications additional indicators to assess the possibility of lung transplantation are: continued lung deterioration despite optimal medical therapy, successful smoking cessation, application of maximal pharmacological treatment, long-term rehabilitation and oxygen therapy and application of previous surgical treatment. After transplantation, the individual usually experiences an improvement in exercise capacity, lung function, and quality of life (SILVA, 2015).

Non-pharmacological therapy is based on pulmonary rehabilitation, the use of oxygen, and surgical interventions. Pulmonary rehabilitation basically includes physical conditioning exercises, nutritional advice and education, with the aim of reducing symptoms, and increasing the patient's participation in his daily activities. Oxygen therapy is the main non-pharmacological treatment used in very severe stages of the disease, and may be used in the long term, during exercise and to relieve dyspnoea crises. Surgical interventions are restricted to patients in very severe stage of the disease, such as in cases of emphysema, in which lung volume reduction surgery and lung transplantation may be indicated (POSADA, 2011).

Physiotherapeutic treatment of patients with COPD aims to increase the capacity to perform the activities of daily living, using exercises that may increase the mobility of the rib cage and the strength of the respiratory muscles, consequently helping to prevent the occurrence of respiratory infections. Exercises aimed at increasing the mobility of the rib cage improve chest expansion, quality of life, and submaximal exercise capacity, reducing dyspnea and depression levels (RODRIGUES, 2012).

Regarding the training with upper limbs, SBPT (2000) recommends the practice of these activities with weights, sticks, or elastic bands in order to minimize dyspnea. Some shoulder muscles assist breathing, and when involved in other activities, these muscles have a diminished function in breathing, increasing the work of the diaphragm. Muscle strengthening is recommended because of exercise intolerance due to muscle weakness in individuals with COPD, affecting mainly the lower limbs (FERREIRA, 2010).

Malnutrition is a significant problem in COPD patients. Therefore, in this population at risk, nutritional depletion and changes in body composition are independent and strong predictors of mortality. Malnutrition is often associated with anaemia, susceptibility to infections and loss of muscle mass, worsening dyspnoea and limiting exercise capacity. BMI is an independent prognostic factor in COPD patients. A decrease in BMI is associated with increased mortality and risk of developing COPD. An increase in BMI may even improve lung function in COPD patients. COPD patients who are underweight or who experience weight loss during follow-up should be offered nutritional supplement therapy. However, the long-term benefits of nutritional supplementation are still to be determined (SILVA, 2015).

CONCLUDING REMARKS

The chronic obstructive pulmonary disease that deserves attention from health professionals, as well as from rulers and society. It is a chronic, progressive disease that, despite being preventable, has been very frequent in Brazil and worldwide, due to both the change in the epidemiological profile and the high rates of smoking, a very important risk factor for the development of COPD.

The diagnosis of the disease is considerably simple, being made from the classification provided by the clinical history of the patient, together with spirometry tests and chest X-ray when necessary. The clinical symptomatology is characterised by dyspnoea, cough and expectoration. The condition may worsen with the association of other elements which increase inflammation, such as viruses, bacteria and fungus. Among the complications of the disease are bronchitis, obstructive bronchiolitis, pulmonary emphysema and even insufficiency in some cases. Physical disability is a factor that can make it difficult for the carrier to live with the disease.

As with other treatments, some patients may be resistant and even choose not to adhere. It is important that a significant work of explanation is done for patients and family members, especially regarding lifestyle changes and drug and non-drug therapy. The ability of health professionals is essential to promote this information and consequently a better assistance.

Therefore, in view of the above, it is possible to infer that much still needs to be studied about this disease. New studies must be conducted in order to fill in the gaps that persist with respect to diagnosis and treatment. Thus, it will be possible to develop increasingly efficient treatment techniques that promote quality of life for COPD patients.

REFERENCES

ALVES, D. A. **Investigation of the correspondence between crackling sound indices and respiratory impedance in COPD**. Dissertation (Master in Electrical Engineering) - Federal University of Santa Catarina, Florianópolis, 2014.

ALVES, D. M. R. **Chronic obstructive pulmonary disease**. Dissertation (Integrated Master in Medicine) - Faculty of Health Sciences, Portugal, 2019.

AZAMBUJA, R., et al. Overview of chronic obstructive pulmonary disease. **Revista Hospital Universitário Pedro Ernesto**, [S.I.], v. 12, n. 2, jun. 2013. ISSN 19832567. Disponívelem :
https://www.e-publicacoes.uerj.br/index.php/revistahupe/article/view/8483/6302. Accessed on: 23 jan. 2021.

BARTHOLO, R. M. Clinical differences between asthma and chronic obstructive pulmonary disease. **Revista Hospital Universitário Pedro Ernesto**, v. 12, n. 2, jun. 2013. Disponívelem :
https://www.e-publicacoes.uerj.br/index.php/revistahupe/article/view/8488/6311. Accessed on: 26 jan. 2021.

COSTA, C. H; RUFINO, R. Treatment of chronic obstructive pulmonary disease. **Revista HUPE**, Rio de Janeiro, v. 12, n. 2, abril/jun., 2013.

COSTA, D. I. S. **Normas de Orientação Clínica na abordagem da DPOC**. Dissertation (Integrated Master's Degree in Medicine) - Faculty of Medicine of the University of Porto, 2010.

COSTA, L. D. **V. Lymphocyte populations in chronic obstructive pulmonary disease (COPD): study of peripheral blood cells and literature review**. Dissertation (Master in Biomedical Sciences) - Universidade da Beira Interior, 2014. Available at: https://ubibliorum.ubi.pt/handle/10400.6/5672. Accessed: 02 Jan. 2021.

DUMKE, A. **Effects of Proprioceptive Neuromuscular Facilitation Applied to the Accessory Musculature of Respiration on Pulmonary Variables and Muscle Activation in Patients with COPD**. Dissertation (PhD in Pulmonary Sciences) - Federal University of Rio Grande do Sul, Porto Alegre, 2012.

ESPANHOL, R. L. P. COPD - **Chronic Obstructive Pulmonary Disease**. Dissertation (Master's in Pharmaceutical Sciences) - Fernando Pessoa University, 2011. Available at: https://bdigital.ufp.pt/handle/10284/2462. Accessed on: 27 Jan. 2021.

FARIAS, G. M. S. **Qualidade de vida da pessoa com DPOC**. Dissertation (Master's Degree in Rehabilitation Nursing) - Escola Superior de Saúde do Viseu, Portugal, 2011.

FERNANDES, S. R. C. **Early Diagnosis and Treatment of COPD, Contributions from Rehabilitation Nursing**. Dissertation (Master's Degree in Rehabilitation Nursing) - Escola Superior de Saúde, Portugal, 2019.

FERREIRA, D. S. A. **Physiological and functional changes in people with COPD, in acute phase, after the implementation of active resisted exercises of the upper limbs**. Dissertation (Master's Degree in Rehabilitation Nursing) - Escola Superior de Saúde de Bragança, 2014. Available at: https://bibliotecadigital.ipb.pt/handle/10198/10437. Access on: 02 Jan. 2021.

FERREIRA, V. C. **Functional Independence of the Elderly with Chronic Obstructive Pulmonary Disease**. Dissertation (Master of Science) - Nursing School of Ribeirão Preto of the University of São Paulo, São Paulo, 2010.

GIL, L. C; FREITAS, S; CORDEIRO, C. R. **Clinical phenotypes of COPD**. Dissertation (Master in Medicine in the scientific area of Pulmonology) - Faculty of Medicine of the University of Coimbra, Portugal, 2013.

GONÇALVES, J. R. **Doença obstrutiva grave = similaridades e diferenças em pacientes portadores de doença pulmonar obstrutiva crônica (DPOC) e/ou bronquiectasias**. Dissertation (Master's in Clinical Medicine) - State University of Campinas, Campinas, 2010. Available at: http://repositorio.unicamp.br/handle/REPOSIP/309664. Accessed on: 01 Jan. 2021.

GUYTON, A. C; HALL, J. E. **Fundamentos de fisiologia médica**. 13. ed. Rio de Janeiro: Elsevier, 2017.

IKE, D., et al. Effects of upper limb resistance exercise on peripheral muscle strength and functional capacity of patient with COPD. **Fisioterapia do Movimento**, Curitiba, v. 23, n.3, p. 429-437, Sep.,

2010. Disponível em: https://www.scielo.br/scielo.php?pid=S0103-5150201000300010&script=sci abstract&tlng=pt#:~:text=INTRODU%C3%87%C3%83O%3A%20A%20disfun%C3%A7%C3%A3o%20muscular%20perif%C3%A9rica,tre inamento%20f%C3%ADsico%20para%20esses%20pacientes. Accessed on: 11 feb. 2021.

LIMA, P. A. L; SANTANA, L. S. R. Alterações **biomecânicas em portadores de doença pulmonar obstrutiva crónica**. Sergipe, 2011.

LOIVOS, L. P. COPD - definitions and concepts - the clinical basis. **Pulmão RJ**, v. 1, n.1,2019.

MACHADO, D. C., et al. Radiological diagnosis of COPD. **Pulmão RJ**, v. 22, n. 2, 2013.

MARCOS, L., et al. Classification of chronic obstructive pulmonary disease by chest radiography. **Revista Radiologia Brasileira**, São Paulo, v. 46, n. 6, p. 327332, dec. 2013. Available at: https://www.scielo.br/scielo.php?pid=S0100-398420130006003278&script=sciarttext&tlng=en. Accessed on: 26 Jan. 2021.

MARCHIORI, R. C., et al. Diagnosis and treatment of exacerbated COPD in the emergency department. **Revista da AMRIGS**, Porto Alegre, 54 (2): 214-223, abr./jun., 2010.

MARQUES, M. A. T. **Systemic repercussions of COPD**. Dissertation (PhD in Health Sciences) - Faculty of Medicine, University of Coimbra, Coimbra, 2014.

MELO, L. P; BATISTA, A. N; JUNIOR, J. F. L. Chronic obstructive pulmonary disease in the elderly: Brazilian epidemiological profile between 2012 and 2016. *In:* Congresso Internacional de Envelhecimento Humano, 2016, Rio Grande do Sul. **Annals...**Rio Grande do Sul: UPF, 2016.

MOORE, K. L; DALEY II, A. F. **Anatomia orientada para a clínica**. 7a edição. Guanabara Koogan, Rio de Janeiro, 2014.

PASCHOAL, I. A; MOREIRA, M. M. Physiopathogenesis (and Immunology) of Chronic Obstructive Pulmonary Disease (COPD). **Paulista Pulmonology**, v. 29, n. 3, São Paulo, 2016.

PEREIRA, A. C. A. C. **Factors associated with postural balance alteration and prediction of falls in patients with chronic**

obstructive pulmonary disease. Dissertation (Master of Science) - University of São Paulo School of Medicine, São Paulo, 2017. Available at: https://www.teses.usp.br/teses/disponiveis/5/5160/tde-23042018-115127/en.php. Accessed on: 11 feb. 2021.

POSADA, W. A. **Doença pulmonar obstrutiva crônica (DPOC): revisão sobre a relação da educação com a adesão ao tratamento e a qualidade de vida dos pacientes**. 2011. Trabalho de Conclusão de Curso - Faculdade de Farmácia da Universidade Federal do Rio Grande do Sul, Porto Alegre, 2011.

PRESTES, D., et al. Relationship between the risk of dysphagia and health status of individuals with chronic obstructive pulmonary disease. **Communication Disorders, Audiology and Swallowing**, São Paulo, v. 32, n. 4, Sept., 2019. Available from: https://www.scielo.br/scielo.php?pid=S2317-17822020000400309&script=sci arttext. Accessed on: 11 Feb. 2021.

RABAHI, M. F. Epidemiology of COPD: facing challenges. **Pulmão RJ**, Rio de Janeiro, v. 22, n. 2, p. 4-8, 2013.

RUFINO, R; COSTA, C. H. Pathogenesis of chronic obstructive pulmonary disease. **Revista HUPE**, Rio de Janeiro, v. 12, n. 2, jun. 2013.

ROCHA, S. M. P. **Impact of a respiratory rehabilitation program on the quality of life and activities of daily living of people with chronic obstructive pulmonary disease**. Dissertation (Master's Degree in Rehabilitation Nursing) - Nursing School of Porto, Porto, 2017.

RODRIGUES, C. P., et al. Effect of an exercise program directed to thoracic mobility in COPD. **Fisioterapia em Movimento**, Curitiba, v. 25, n. 2, p. 343-349, abr./jun., 2012. Available at: https://www.scielo.br/scielo.php?pid=S0103-51502012000200012&script=sciarttext. Accessed on: 11 feb. 2021.

ROSA, F. P. **Doença pulmonar obstrutiva crônica e transtorno de de deglutição: revisão de literatura**. Dissertation (Bachelor of Speech Therapy) - Federal University of Santa Catarina, Florianópolis, 2013. Available at: https://repositorio.ufsc.br/handle/123456789/115316. Accessed on: 11 feb. 2021.

SAMPAIO, M. S. **Chronic obstructive pulmonary disease as a risk factor for suicide: A systematic review and meta analysis**. 2019.

Dissertation (Professional Master) - Universidade Estadual de Campinas, Faculdade de Odontologia de Piracicaba, São Paulo, 2019.

SANTOS, I. G. D; SENA, J. T. S; COSTA, A. C. S. M. Respiratory muscle strengthening in patients with chronic obstructive pulmonary disease. **Brazilian Journal of Health Review**, Curitiba, v. 2, n. 2, p. 6, mar./apr., 2019.

SILVA, M. C. C. **Chronic obstructive pulmonary disease in the elderly: non-pharmacological therapy and pulmonary rehabilitation**. Dissertation (Integrated Master's Degree in Medicine) - Faculty of Medicine, University of Coimbra, Coimbra, 2015.

STANDRING, S. **Gray's anatomy: the anatomical basis of clinical practice**. 40a edição. Rio de Janeiro: Elsevier, 2010.

TANDO, A. H. C. **Therapeutic approach to COPD: new strategy**. Dissertation (Integrated Master's Degree in Pharmaceutical Sciences), Porto, 2016. Available at: https://bdigital.ufp.pt/handle/10284/5799. Accessed on: 28 Jan. 2021.

TONIDANDEL, P. R. **Construction and content validation of a questionnaire to identify risk factors for chronic obstructive pulmonary disease**. Dissertation (Master of Science in Clinical Medicine part) - Faculty of Medical Sciences, State University of Campinas, Campinas, 2019.

VIEIRA, R. H. G. **Peripheral and respiratory muscle strength in chronic obstructive pulmonary disease**. 2017. 52f. Dissertation (Master in Physiotherapy) - Health Sciences Center, Federal University of Rio Grande do Norte, Natal, 2017. Available at: https://repositorio.ufrn.br/handle/123456789/24071. Accessed on 11 Feb. 2021.

ZONZIN, G. A., et al. What is important for the diagnosis of COPD? **Pulmão RJ**, Rio de Janeiro, v. 26, n. 1, 2017.

CONTENTS

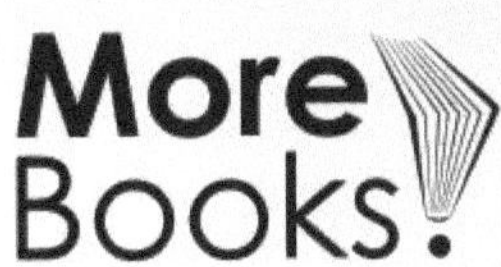

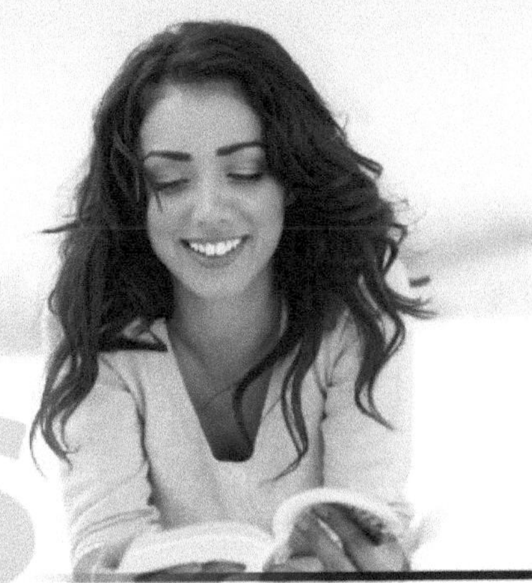

I want morebooks!

Buy your books fast and straightforward online - at one of world's fastest growing online book stores! Environmentally sound due to Print-on-Demand technologies.

Buy your books online at
www.morebooks.shop

Kaufen Sie Ihre Bücher schnell und unkompliziert online – auf einer der am schnellsten wachsenden Buchhandelsplattformen weltweit! Dank Print-On-Demand umwelt- und ressourcenschonend produzi ert.

Bücher schneller online kaufen
www.morebooks.shop

KS OmniScriptum Publishing
Brivibas gatve 197
LV-1039 Riga, Latvia
Telefax: +371 686 204 55

info@omniscriptum.com
www.omniscriptum.com

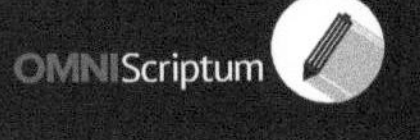

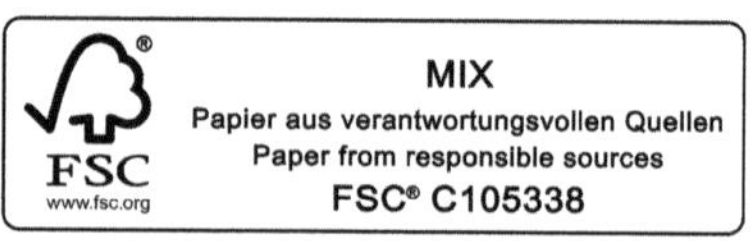

Printed by Books on Demand GmbH, Norderstedt / Germany